COPD DIET

COOKBOOK

Boost Lung Health, Reduce Inflammation, And Enhance Breathing With Easy, Low-Sodium Meals

DR ELIAN GRIFFIN

DISCLAIMER

The nutritional recommendations and recipes in this book are meant solely for informative reasons. They are not meant to replace the counsel, diagnosis, or care of a qualified medical expert. If you have any doubts about a medical condition or dietary requirements, you should always see your physician or another trained healthcare expert.

All reasonable efforts have been taken by the author and publisher to ensure that the information contained in this book is correct as of the date of publication. Recommendations may alter, though, as medical knowledge is always changing. When using any of the recipes or instructions found here, the user assumes all liability and assumes no risk, whether personal or otherwise. People who have certain dietary requirements or medical issues should speak with a healthcare provider for personalized guidance. The given recipes are only ideas; you may need to adjust them to suit your own nutritional needs, tastes, and tolerances.

When you use this book, you agree to release the publisher, the author, and their representatives from any liability for any claims, damages, liabilities, costs, or expenditures resulting from your use of the book.

TABLE OF CONTENTS

ABOUT THE BOOK

The "COPD Diet Cookbook" is an invaluable tool for anyone coping with the difficulties of having Chronic Obstructive Pulmonary Disease (COPD). Its significance stems from the understanding that nutrition is critical to managing COPD successfully. This thorough manual starts by outlining the significant effects of COPD on nutritional requirements, highlighting how the illness affects metabolism and raises energy expenditure, making dietary modifications necessary for preserving health and controlling symptoms.

Comprehending the intricacies of COPD is crucial, particularly its diverse range of symptoms and how they affect dietary needs. The cookbook outlines specific objectives: to offer nutrient-dense, easily accessible recipes that are customized to meet the needs of COPD patients, guaranteeing that meals promote respiratory health and general well-being. Organized for ease of use, the book provides direction on making the most of its content, including suggestions for modifying recipes to suit specific dietary preferences and restrictions.

The book provides a foundational understanding of the disease by outlining its symptoms and the critical role that nutrition plays in managing them. It also outlines essential nutrients that are critical for patients with COPD and provides dietary guidelines that are intended to optimize respiratory function and support overall health.

The sections conclude with practical advice on healthy eating habits that are specific to COPD, ensuring that readers can easily incorporate these guidelines into their daily lives.

The book explores doable strategies for meal preparation and planning that are specific to the needs of COPD patients. From making balanced meal plans to offering advice on grocery shopping and meal prep, each section aims to make it easier for COPD patients to maintain a healthy diet despite the obstacles they face.

The recipes are not only nutrient-dense but also take dietary restrictions into account, providing substitutions and adjustments as needed.

The cookbook's recipe sections are especially interesting and varied, providing heart-healthy and COPD-friendly options for any meal occasion. From healthy and nutrient-dense breakfast ideas to heart-healthy soups, salads, and main dishes, each recipe highlights heart-healthy ingredients, low sodium, and lean proteins.

The addition of plant-based and vegetarian options guarantees dietary inclusivity, meeting a range of dietary preferences without sacrificing nutritional integrity.

Beyond mealtimes, the cookbook covers important topics like staying hydrated, managing dietary obstacles like weight fluctuations and digestive problems, and realistic lifestyle modifications for living with COPD. It promotes holistic wellness by including suggestions for stress reduction, better sleep, and assistance in quitting smoking—a comprehensive strategy meant to improve the quality of life for people with COPD.

Through answering commonly asked questions and providing useful information on meal planning, supplementation, and dietary adjustments, the cookbook further empowers readers with practical insights on managing COPD. This comprehensive investigation guarantees that all facets of nutritional support for COPD patients are addressed, providing not only recipes but a comprehensive manual on living a healthier lifestyle despite the obstacles presented by the disease.

CHAPTER ONE

COPD DIET INTRODUCTION

IMPORTANT OF COPD DIET MANAGEMENT

A well-planned diet is critical to the management of COPD (Chronic Obstructive Pulmonary Disease) because it supports overall health and minimizes symptoms. People with COPD frequently have breathing difficulties, which can cause them to lose appetite and energy.

As a result, maintaining strength and controlling weight require a diet high in nutrients. Important objectives include enhancing lung function and avoiding complications like infections and exacerbations.

A diet for people with COPD emphasizes low-energy, easily digested foods that support effective breathing; it also places a strong emphasis on foods high in nutrients, such as fruits, vegetables, whole grains, and lean proteins, which help meet nutritional needs without adding extra calories; drinking enough water is also important to keep mucus thin and reduce coughing.

In addition, a balanced diet can help control other conditions linked to COPD, like heart disease and osteoporosis. It's crucial to watch how much salt you eat to avoid fluid retention and reduce the amount of stress on your heart and lungs. All things considered, a well-managed diet for COPD promotes general health, increases vitality, and improves the quality of life by lowering symptoms and complications.

RECOGNIZING THE EFFECTS OF COPD ON NUTRITION

As a progressive lung disease marked by airflow obstruction and breathing difficulties, COPD is frequently brought on by prolonged exposure to irritants such as pollutants or cigarette smoke. It impairs lung function, making it more difficult to breathe effectively, which can lead to weight loss, muscle weakness, and nutritional deficiencies because of decreased appetite and increased energy expenditure.

To manage the symptoms of COPD and slow down the disease's progression, nutrition is essential. For example, eating enough protein helps repair and strengthen muscles, which is important because COPD can cause muscle atrophy.

Foods high in antioxidants, such as leafy greens and berries, can help reduce inflammation and oxidative stress in the lungs. Finally, maintaining a healthy weight through balanced nutrition can improve overall respiratory function and quality of life.

Comprehending how COPD affects nutrition entails identifying particular dietary requirements and obstacles. For instance, avoiding gas-producing foods can alleviate bloating and discomfort that accompany COPD symptoms. Moreover, certain medications may impact nutrient absorption or metabolism, requiring dietary modifications. In this way, patients with COPD can effectively manage their condition and improve their quality of life by customizing their nutrition.

The COPD Diet Cookbook's main objective is to empower COPD patients and caregivers with reachable meal options that support overall wellness and effectively manage symptoms by offering practical guidance and recipes that are specific to the nutritional needs of people with COPD. These recipes are easy to prepare, high in nutrients, and focused on improving respiratory health.

The cookbook not only supports lung health but also aims to inform readers about the role that certain nutrients play in the management of COPD. It highlights foods high in antioxidants, omega-3 fatty acids, and vitamins that support immune system function and lung function. By including these foods in daily meals, people with COPD can improve their nutritional intake and quality of life.

In addition, the cookbook is a useful tool for preparing tasty meals that adhere to the dietary restrictions that are typical in the management of COPD.

These include low-sodium, high-fiber, and easily digestible options that reduce digestive strain and maximize nutrient absorption. In the end, the COPD Diet Cookbook aims to promote overall health, improve respiratory function, and improve quality of life by offering wholesome and delectable meal options.

HOW TO MAKE THE MOST OF THIS BOOK

To make the most of the COPD Diet Cookbook, you should first become acquainted with its layout and contents. Read through the introductory sections to gain an understanding of the fundamentals of managing COPD with nutrition, as well as the nutritional objectives listed for each recipe and how they relate to reducing symptoms and enhancing general health.

Then, look through the recipe sections, which are categorized by meal type or nutritional focus. Each recipe has comprehensive instructions, ingredient lists, and nutritional data to help you make an informed decision.

You can also modify recipes to suit your dietary requirements and preferences by using the tips that are included in them. For example, you can change the portion sizes or substitute ingredients to accommodate food allergies or intolerances.

Whether you're using the cookbook's suggested meal plans or incorporating recipes into your current meal rotation, meal planning can be made easier by making meals in bulk to save time and effort—especially on days when managing your symptoms may be more difficult. With careful attention to the guidelines and tips offered, you can successfully incorporate the COPD Diet Cookbook into your daily routine to support respiratory health and optimal nutrition.

ADVICE ON TAILORING RECIPES TO SPECIFIC REQUIREMENTS

By customizing the recipes in the COPD Diet Cookbook to your unique needs, you can be sure that every meal supports your unique health goals and preferences.

To start, go over the nutritional information and ingredient list of each recipe, making note of any ingredients that might need to be substituted because of intolerances, allergies, or personal preferences; for instance, you can change the seasoning to suit your taste preferences or swap out dairy for non-dairy alternatives.

To effectively control calorie intake and manage the symptoms of COPD, pay attention to portion sizes. You may also want to divide recipes into smaller servings or change the quantities of ingredients to achieve the nutritional requirements you require without going overboard.

Lastly, you may want to try different cooking techniques to maximize flavor and nutrient retention without going overboard with your dietary restrictions.

You can enjoy tasty meals that improve lung function and quality of life by tailoring recipes in the COPD Diet Cookbook. Speak with a healthcare provider or registered dietitian for personalized advice on modifying recipes to your unique COPD management plan. They can offer insights into nutrient requirements, portion control, and dietary adjustments that support respiratory health and overall well-being.

CHAPTER TWO

ESSENTIALS OF COPD AND DIET

AN OVERVIEW OF THE SYMPTOMS OF COPD

The progressive lung disease known as Chronic Obstructive Pulmonary Disease (COPD) is characterized by a restriction of airflow that makes breathing difficult. The disease can greatly affect daily activities such as walking and climbing stairs. It is commonly brought on by long-term exposure to irritants such as cigarette smoke, pollutants, or genetic factors.

Effective management of COPD depends on early diagnosis. Spirometry tests are used by medical professionals to measure lung function and evaluate the severity of COPD based on symptoms and exacerbations. Treatment aims to reduce symptoms, enhance quality of life, and prevent complications using medication, pulmonary rehabilitation, and lifestyle modifications.

A balanced diet can help COPD patients maintain a healthy weight, strengthen respiratory muscles, and boost immune function to prevent infections. Adequate nutrition also aids in energy conservation, which is crucial for individuals with COPD who often expend more energy on breathing. Nutrition plays a pivotal role in managing COPD by supporting overall health and minimizing symptoms.

Nutritionists advise small, frequent meals to prevent bloating and breathing discomfort, as large meals can put pressure on the diaphragm and lungs.

Patients with COPD should concentrate on consuming nutrient-dense foods rich in vitamins, minerals, and antioxidants. These include fruits, vegetables, whole grains, lean proteins, and healthy fats. Appropriate hydration is essential to keep mucus thin and easier to cough up, reducing the risk of respiratory infections.

Given their roles in immune system function and respiratory health, several nutrients are especially helpful for COPD patients: antioxidants like vitamins C and E protect lung tissue from oxidative stress caused by free radicals, a common cause of COPD; vitamin D supports immune system function and may lessen exacerbations in COPD patients deficient in this vitamin; omega-3 fatty acids found in fish like salmon or flaxseeds help reduce inflammation in the lungs and may improve lung function.

Foods like lean meats, poultry, beans, and dairy products provide high-quality protein essential for muscle repair and energy. Fiber-rich foods like whole grains, fruits, and vegetables aid in digestion and help regulate blood sugar levels, promoting stable energy throughout the day for COPD patients managing fatigue. Protein is crucial for maintaining muscle strength, especially respiratory muscles, which can weaken in COPD.

Meals should be well-balanced, emphasizing a variety of nutrient-rich foods while limiting sodium and processed sugars that can contribute to inflammation and fluid retention. Portion control is essential to prevent overeating and discomfort that can strain breathing. Patients with COPD benefit from adhering to specific dietary guidelines tailored to manage symptoms and improve overall health.

For stable energy levels and digestive health, choose whole grains like oats, brown rice, and whole wheat bread over refined grains.

Lean proteins like chicken, fish, beans, and tofu should be included to support muscle strength and repair, which is important for COPD patients experiencing muscle wasting. A diet high in fruits and vegetables is ideal because they are low in calories, rich in fiber, and provide essential vitamins and minerals.

It can be difficult to maintain a healthy diet when suffering from COPD, but there are a few doable strategies that can make meal planning and preparation easier. For example, choose to eat smaller, more frequent meals throughout the day to minimize the effort of eating and digestion, which can strain respiratory muscles. You can also prepare meals ahead of time or ask family members to help if you are too tired to cook.

Consider using portable oxygen if prescribed during meal preparation or eating to ensure adequate oxygen intake. Limit caffeine and alcohol as they can dehydrate the body and interfere with medications used to manage COPD symptoms. Stay hydrated by drinking plenty of fluids, preferably water, to keep mucus thin and easier to clear from the airways.

Patients with COPD can support their nutritional needs and improve their overall quality of life by focusing on nutrient-dense snacks like yogurt with fresh fruit, nuts, or whole-grain crackers to maintain energy levels between meals. They can also experiment with herbs and spices to flavor dishes without adding extra salt, which can contribute to fluid retention and worsen symptoms.

CHAPTER THREE

MEAL PLANNING FOR COPD DIET

MAKING A MEAL PLAN THAT IS BALANCED

When creating a balanced meal plan for COPD (chronic obstructive pulmonary disease), the emphasis should be on nutrient-dense foods that promote respiratory health and overall well-being. To start, include a range of vitamin- and antioxidant-rich fruits and vegetables, such as citrus fruits, berries, and leafy greens; these foods help strengthen lung function and reduce inflammation; whole grains, such as brown rice and quinoa, offer sustained energy without causing excessive discomfort or bloating; and lean proteins, like chicken, fish, and legumes, are crucial for preserving immune function and maintaining muscle strength.

A well-rounded diet that prioritizes nutrient-rich foods can help people with COPD manage their condition and enhance their overall quality of life. Beyond these basic components, it's important to take into account healthy fats like avocados, nuts, and olive oil, which provide essential fatty acids that aid in reducing inflammation and supporting heart health. Finally, avoiding processed foods high in trans fats and sugars is important to prevent exacerbation of COPD symptoms. Finally, staying hydrated by drinking plenty of water throughout the day helps thin mucus and ease breathing difficulties.

MEAL TIMING AND PORTION MANAGEMENT

To manage the symptoms of COPD and optimize nutritional intake, portion control, and timing are critical. Start with mindful eating, emphasizing smaller, more frequent meals instead of large ones. This helps avoid bloating and discomfort and ensures a steady supply of nutrients throughout the day. Eating slowly and thoroughly chewing food is beneficial as well as reducing the strain on respiratory function.

Meal timing: Aim for a balanced distribution of carbohydrates, proteins, and fats in each meal to support sustained energy and muscle function.

Including snacks between meals, like yogurt with fresh fruit or whole-grain crackers with hummus, can help maintain blood sugar levels and prevent energy dips. Eating at regular intervals can also help maintain stable energy levels and prevent overeating.

Eating lighter meals in the evening can promote better sleep quality and digestive comfort. Individuals with COPD can improve their nutritional intake and general well-being by practicing portion control, mindful eating, and strategic meal timing. It's also important to think about when to schedule meals daily activities and medication schedules.

GUIDELINES FOR COPD PATIENTS WHEN GROCERY

For people with COPD, navigating the grocery store can be intimidating, but with a little preparation, it can become a manageable task. Begin by making a shopping list based on your balanced meal plan, emphasizing whole grains, fresh produce, lean proteins, and healthy fats.

This way, you can make sure you have wholesome ingredients on hand and avoid making impulsive purchases of less healthful items.

Prioritize items that are simple to prepare and don't take a lot of time to cook. Convenient options that cut down on preparation time while still providing essential nutrients are pre-cut vegetables, canned beans, and frozen fruits. When choosing canned goods and packaged foods, go for low-sodium options to help control blood pressure and fluid retention—two issues that can be common for people with COPD.

With these grocery shopping tips, people with COPD can streamline their shopping experiences and maintain a healthy diet to support their health goals. Firstly, think about shopping during off-peak hours to avoid crowds and reduce exposure to respiratory irritants. Secondly, use grocery delivery or curbside pickup services if available to minimize physical exertion and conserve energy. Lastly, be mindful of perishable items and plan your meals for the week to minimize food waste.

Meal prepping is an effective way for people with COPD to make cooking easier daily and guarantee that they always have access to nutritious meals. To begin, set aside a certain day each week to plan and cook meals ahead of time.

Make your meal selections from recipes that are simple to batch-cook and portion into individual servings, like casseroles, soups, and stews. Once your meals are ready, store them in freezer or refrigerator containers so that you always have access to wholesome options throughout the week.

When meal prepping, think about including ingredients that can be used in several different dishes, like quinoa, roasted vegetables, and grilled chicken. To ensure food safety and quality, label containers with the date of preparation and instructions for reheating. Include snacks like chopped fruits, yogurt cups, and almonds in your meal prep routine to keep your energy up between meals.

Meal prep can be made more efficient and enjoyable by delegating tasks or involving family members in the process. By implementing these meal prep strategies, people with COPD can save time, and energy, and maintain a consistent supply of nutrient-dense meals to support their health and well-being. Simplify cooking tasks by using kitchen tools and appliances like rice cookers, slow cookers, and food processors.

MODIFYING RECIPES TO MEET DIETARY REQUIREMENTS

For people with COPD who may have particular nutritional requirements or food sensitivities, it is critical to modify recipes to accommodate dietary restrictions.

Begin by identifying common allergens or intolerances, such as gluten, dairy, or specific spices, and select recipes that are simple to modify or substitute. For instance, you can bake recipes that call for wheat flour to be replaced with almond flour or gluten-free flour blends to make gluten-free versions of your favorite treats.

For those who are vegetarians or vegans, think about other protein sources like lentils, tofu, or tempeh. Instead of using dairy products, try plant-based alternatives like almond milk, coconut yogurt, or cashew cheese to minimize lactose intake and promote comfort in the digestive tract. Try seasoning food with herbs and spices to add flavor instead of salt, which can cause fluid retention and aggravate symptoms of COPD.

Recipes can be modified to meet dietary restrictions and preferences, allowing people with COPD to enjoy tasty and nourishing meals that effectively support their health goals. Prioritize nutrient-dense ingredients that support respiratory health and overall well-being. Include plenty of colorful fruits and vegetables, lean proteins, whole grains, and healthy fats to create well-balanced meals. Portion sizes should be considered to prevent overeating and minimize discomfort during digestion.

RICH IN NUTRIENT SMOOTHIES AND SHAKES

Smoothies and shakes that are high in nutrients can be a great way to start your COPD-friendly breakfast routine. They are quick and simple to make, and they contain concentrated doses of vitamins, minerals, and antioxidants that are important for respiratory health. To start, choose antioxidant-rich ingredients like kale, spinach, or berries, which help fight inflammation and oxidative stress in the lungs. Then, add a source of protein like Greek yogurt or protein powder to support muscle repair and strength. Finally, add ingredients like chia seeds or flaxseeds for their omega-3 fatty acids, which can help reduce inflammation and improve lung function.

Smooth and creamy smoothies can be made by simply blending your chosen ingredients with a liquid base, like almond milk or coconut water until the consistency is desired; if you prefer a shake, blend ingredients with a protein-rich liquid, like soy milk or dairy milk, and taste it; experiment with different combinations to find flavors that suit your palate while still meeting your nutritional requirements. These refreshing smoothies and shakes are a great way to increase your intake of nutrients and support your overall health.

Nutrient-dense smoothies and shakes can be a game-changer for sustaining energy levels and promoting respiratory health. By carefully selecting ingredients and blending them into delectable beverages, you can start your day with a dose of vitamins, minerals, and antioxidants necessary for lung function.

Whether you prefer the convenience of a smoothie or the protein boost of a shake, these breakfast options provide a tasty and useful way to support your nutritional goals. You can experiment with different combinations of ingredients and flavors to find combinations that appeal to your palate while offering vital nutrients to support your respiratory health.

Energizing breakfast bowls that support your COPD diet can help you start your day off right with a balanced combination of nutrients that support lung health and maintain your energy levels throughout the day. To start, base your bowl with whole grains like quinoa or oats, which provide complex carbohydrates for sustained energy release without spiking blood sugar levels. Then, add a variety of colorful fruits, like citrus fruits, bananas, or berries, which are high in antioxidants and vitamin C and can help reduce inflammation in the lungs. Finally, add nuts or seeds, like almonds, walnuts, or chia seeds, for extra protein and healthy fats that support muscle repair and strength.

To make a breakfast bowl, cook your chosen grains as directed on the package and let them cool slightly. Then, layer your ingredients in a bowl, starting with the grains as the base and adding fruits, nuts, and seeds for flavor and texture. Finally, drizzle with honey or Greek yogurt for extra sweetness and protein.

These breakfast bowls look good and provide a filling and nutritious start to the day. You can adjust the recipe to fit your dietary requirements and taste preferences while still getting the nutrients you need to support respiratory health.

Breakfast bowls are a flexible and easy way to start your day on a nutritious note. Try experimenting with different combinations of grains, fruits, and nuts to find flavors you love and make sure you get the nutritional support your body needs to thrive. By adding energizing breakfast bowls to your COPD-friendly diet, you can maximize your nutritional intake and support lung function. These bowls are full of vitamins, minerals, and antioxidants that promote overall well-being while providing sustained energy throughout the morning.

OPTIONS FOR HIGH-PROTEIN BREAKFASTS

A complete protein source, eggs can be prepared in a variety of ways, such as scrambled, poached, or as an omelet with vegetables like spinach, tomatoes, or mushrooms.

Eggs also provide essential amino acids necessary for maintaining muscle mass and supporting overall health. Greek yogurt, topped with nuts, seeds, and a drizzle of honey, is another delicious and nutritious high-protein breakfast option that supports your COPD diet. Protein is essential for muscle strength and repair, which is crucial for individuals managing respiratory conditions.

Legumes, which are high in protein and fiber and can help stabilize blood sugar levels and support digestive health, are a great option for plant-based eaters. You can also combine cottage cheese with fresh fruit or whole-grain toast for a balanced breakfast that provides both protein and carbohydrates.

These high-protein breakfast options not only keep you feeling full and satisfied but also provide the necessary nutrients to support respiratory function and overall well-being.

If you include high-protein breakfast options in your COPD-friendly diet, you can be sure that you are getting the essential nutrients required to support overall health and muscle strength. These options are flexible and can be tailored to your specific dietary needs and taste preferences. Whether you prefer plant-based alternatives like legumes and nuts or animal-based alternatives like eggs and dairy, there are many delicious options to try. Start your day off right with a high-protein breakfast that supports respiratory health and fuels your body.

IDEAS FOR QUICK AND SIMPLE BREAKFASTS

Make your morning routine more efficient by incorporating these quick and easy breakfast ideas that are ideal for people with COPD. These options are made to be easily prepared and offer vital nutrients to support respiratory health and overall well-being. To start, try whole grain toast with avocado slices on top and a sprinkle of seeds, like chia or sunflower seeds. Avocado is high in fiber and healthy fats, which help you feel full and satisfied while also supporting digestive health. Another quick option is a smoothie made with frozen fruits, spinach, and a protein-rich liquid like almond milk or yogurt for a nutrient-dense, refreshing breakfast on the go.

You can also make a batch of homemade granola with oats, nuts, and seeds, and add a little honey or maple syrup for sweetness. Serve with milk or yogurt and fresh fruit for a crunchy and filling breakfast option. These quick and easy breakfast ideas can be tailored to your taste preferences and dietary needs, ensuring you start your day with a nutritious and delicious meal. For a savory twist, prepare overnight oats by combining oats with milk or yogurt, chia seeds, and your favorite fruits or nuts in a jar. Refrigerate overnight, and in the morning, you'll have a ready-to-eat breakfast that doesn't require any cooking.

Whether you prefer a simple toast with avocado, a nutrient-packed smoothie, or a make-ahead overnight oats recipe, there are plenty of delicious and nutritious options to explore. By starting your day with a balanced breakfast, you can fuel your body with the nutrients it needs to support respiratory function and overall wellness. These quick and easy breakfast ideas can be incorporated into your COPD-friendly diet and allow you to prioritize your health without sacrificing convenience.

SOME QUICK BREAKFAST IDEAS

Convenience without sacrificing nutrition is the key to making sure you start your day with a nutritious and filling meal. To start, make grab-and-go options such as premade smoothie packs that include frozen fruits, spinach, and individual servings of protein powder; simply blend with liquid in the morning for a quick and nutrient-dense breakfast. Alternatively, prepare overnight oats in portable jars the night before by layering oats, milk or yogurt, fruits, and nuts; pick them up from the refrigerator in the morning for a ready-to-eat meal.

Consider batch-cooking breakfast items like egg muffins loaded with vegetables or homemade granola bars that can be stored in the freezer and reheated or eaten cold when needed.

These make-ahead options save time and ensure you have a nutritious breakfast ready to enjoy even on hectic mornings. By planning and using these helpful tips, you can maintain a healthy breakfast routine that supports your COPD management while accommodating your busy lifestyle. Invest in portable containers or bento boxes that allow you to pack breakfast items like hard-boiled eggs, whole grain muffins, or fruit slices for easy transport.

Whether you prefer portable smoothies, overnight oats, or pre-packed containers with a variety of breakfast items, there are plenty of options to suit your taste and schedule. By prioritizing convenience and nutrition, you can ensure that you start your day with a balanced meal that fuels your body and supports your overall well-being. Implement these tips into your routine to make breakfast on-the-go a seamless part of your COPD-friendly diet. Breakfast on the go doesn't have to be complicated or unhealthy.

SOUPS MADE AT HOME TO BOOST NUTRIENTS

Making your soups is a great way to increase your intake of nutrients while also enjoying delicious flavors. To start, choose seasonal, fresh vegetables and lean proteins such as chicken or beans. To start, make a flavorful base by sautéing onions and garlic in olive oil until fragrant. Next, add chopped vegetables - carrots, celery, and bell peppers - and let them soften. Next, pour in low-sodium broth or water and bring to a simmer. Finally, add herbs - bay leaves, thyme, rosemary, or sage.

To add even more nutrition, you may want to blend part of the soup to get a creamy texture without using a lot of heavy cream. This will keep the fiber and vitamins in the soup and still have a satisfying consistency. Season to taste with salt and pepper, and then add a squeeze of lemon juice or a sprinkle of fresh herbs for a fresh taste. Serve hot and top with a drizzle of olive oil or a dollop of Greek yogurt for extra flavor.

With their ability to provide vital nutrients without being heavy, light and refreshing salads are ideal for a diet aimed at people with COPD. Begin with a base of fresh leafy greens, such as kale, spinach, or arugula; add a variety of colorful vegetables, such as tomatoes, cucumbers, and bell peppers, for flavor and texture; add fruits, such as citrus segments or berries, for a burst of sweetness and extra vitamins; and for added protein, consider grilled chicken breast, boiled eggs, or chickpeas.

Toss the salad gently to coat evenly, ensuring every bite is flavorful. Sprinkle with nuts or seeds for added crunch and healthy fats. Serve right away to preserve freshness and nutrients. Light and refreshing salads are not only nutritious but also simple to prepare, making them a perfect choice for a quick and satisfying meal. Keep dressings light by using olive oil and vinegar or a citrus-based vinaigrette.

Maintaining muscle strength and supporting general health in people with COPD requires a diet high in protein, such as salads made with grilled salmon, tuna, or tofu. Cook the protein to perfection and allow it to cool slightly before adding it to the salad. Mix the protein with different vegetables, such as leafy greens, cherry tomatoes, and sliced avocado, for a balanced meal.

Add whole grains, such as quinoa or barley, for extra fiber and complex carbohydrates. Drizzle with Greek yogurt, lemon juice, and herb dressing for a tangy kick without heavy cream.

Gently toss to mix all ingredients and make sure every bite is full of flavor and protein. High-protein salads are a great option for people with COPD because they help sustain energy levels and support muscle function.

A few easy tips will let you enjoy creamy soups without heavy cream. To start, start with vegetables, like potatoes or cauliflower, which will blend into a creamy texture when sautéed in olive oil until fragrant and golden. Next, add chopped vegetables and cook until softened; pour in water or low-sodium broth; simmer until vegetables are tender; and finally, blend with an immersion blender or food processor until smooth.

Creamy soups without heavy cream are a delicious and nutritious option for those with COPD, providing comfort and satisfaction without compromising health. To add extra richness, stir in a small amount of Greek yogurt or low-fat milk right before serving.

This adds creaminess without the heaviness of traditional cream, while still providing protein and calcium. Season with herbs and spices like paprika, parsley, or thyme to enhance flavor without adding extra calories.

To make soups and salads more enjoyable and fulfilling, start with aromatic vegetables (onions, garlic, and celery work well as a base for soups), which you can sauté in olive oil until fragrant and softened, releasing their natural flavors. Then, add fresh herbs (like basil, cilantro, or dill) to give your dishes more depth and complexity.

Achieve a harmony of flavors and textures in your salads by experimenting with different combinations of fruits, vegetables, and proteins. Toss in some nuts or seeds for a nutty crunch and add flavor before adding them to salads.

Use a range of spices and seasonings, such as cumin, ginger, or smoked paprika, to create interesting and delectable dishes.

With a little creativity and attention to detail, you can make soups and salads that are both nutritious and delicious, ideal for supporting your health and well-being. By focusing on using fresh, high-quality ingredients and experimenting with different flavors to find combinations that you enjoy, you can easily elevate the flavor of your soups and salads while adhering to a COPD-friendly diet.

HEALTHY SIDE DISHES FOR WELL-ROUNDED MEALS

For COPD patients, a balanced diet should include healthy sides that enhance main meals without negatively impacting respiratory health. Choose sides that are high in fiber, vitamins, and minerals, and avoid sodium and saturated fats. For starters, try simple vegetable sides like steamed broccoli or spinach, which are low in calories and high in antioxidants. Roasted sweet potatoes, on the other hand, provide fiber and potassium, which support overall lung function. If you prefer grains, quinoa salads with colorful vegetables and light vinaigrette offer protein and complex carbohydrates that are necessary for sustained energy levels.

Bean salads and hummus with whole-grain crackers are two examples of protein-rich side dishes that help sustain the muscle strength required for breathing. These dishes are also simple to make and can be refrigerated for easy access during meal times.

Brown rice pilaf with mixed vegetables or lentil soup is two heartier side options that offer a balance of carbohydrates and protein without being too heavy on the digestive tract. By emphasizing nutrient-dense options, patients with COPD can improve their overall diet while supporting respiratory health through well-balanced side dishes.

IDEAS FOR CARRY-ALONG SNACKS FOR COPD PATIENTS

To sustain energy levels throughout the day, COPD patients should have easy-to-transport, portable snack options. Try fresh fruit slices or pre-cut vegetables with hummus, which are high in fiber and vitamins and easy to digest. These snacks can be packed in small containers or zip-lock bags for portability when traveling or on-the-go. Another option is yogurt with granola or nuts, which are high in protein and calcium and easy on the stomach.

Trail mix, which combines nuts, seeds, and dried fruit, is a good source of healthy fats, protein, and carbohydrates for those who need a quick energy boost.

Snacking shouldn't be done with high sodium or saturated fats because these can worsen symptoms; instead, opt for low-sodium snacks like air-popped popcorn or whole-grain crackers with cheese for a filling snack that won't damage respiratory health. COPD patients can effectively manage their condition by planning ahead of time and preparing these portable snacks.

OPTIONS FOR LOW-CALORIE SNACKING

Maintaining a healthy weight and supporting overall respiratory function can be achieved by including low-calorie snacks in a diet for people with COPD. Low-calorie, high-vitamin fresh fruit, like apples or berries, can be eaten on their own or combined with a small amount of yogurt or cottage cheese for extra protein and calcium. Low-calorie, low-fiber vegetable sticks, like carrots or celery with a light dip, are a great way to satisfy cravings in between meals.

Snacking should be nutrient-dense and support energy levels without causing digestive discomfort.

Low-calorie snacks like unsalted almonds or a small serving of whole-grain cereal with skim milk can provide sustained energy without the added calories from sugar or fat. A healthy diet and respiratory health can be supported by choosing low-calorie options for COPD patients. A savory option to consider is rice cakes topped with avocado or lean turkey slices, which offer a balance of carbohydrates and protein while being low in calories.

RECIPES FOR SEASONAL AND FRESH SNACKS

Fresh and seasonal ingredients add flavor vital nutrients and antioxidants to snack recipes for people with COPD. For a savory option, try making a salsa with fresh tomatoes, onions, and cilantro, served with whole-grain tortilla chips for extra fiber. Seasonal fruits like watermelon or berries are also refreshing and high in vitamins C and A, which support immune function and respiratory health. You can eat these fruits on their own or blend them into smoothies with low-fat yogurt or almond milk for a creamy, nutritious treat.

Soups made from seasonal vegetables like butternut squash or pumpkin offer warmth and comfort while providing essential nutrients like beta-carotene and fiber. By experimenting with fresh and seasonal snack recipes, COPD patients can enjoy a variety of flavors while supporting their respiratory health through nutritious ingredients. Salads with seasonal vegetables like cucumbers, bell peppers, and leafy greens provide a mix of vitamins and minerals while being light on the stomach. Dress salads with a homemade vinaigrette made from olive oil and vinegar for a flavorful yet healthful option.

ADVICE ON NUTRITIOUS SNACKING PRACTICES

For COPD patients, maintaining energy levels and supporting overall well-being requires developing healthy snacking habits. To start, prepare snacks in advance and portion them into small containers or zip-lock bags for convenient access. This helps prevent impulsive eating and guarantees that snacks are balanced and nutritious.

Select snacks that are low in saturated fats and sodium and high in fiber, vitamins, and protein, such as Greek yogurt with fresh fruit, whole-grain crackers with hummus, or a handful of nuts and seeds.

Adopting these healthy snacking habits can help COPD patients maintain a balanced diet and effectively support their respiratory health. Sugary snacks and beverages should be avoided because they can spike blood sugar levels and lead to weight gain, which can exacerbate COPD symptoms. Instead, choose snacks that provide sustained energy without the added sugars, like fresh fruit, vegetables, or whole-grain cereals. Dehydration can also exacerbate respiratory symptoms, so it's important to stay hydrated throughout the day by drinking plenty of water or herbal teas.

TIPS FOR HYDRATION FOR PEOPLE WITH COPD

Because COPD patients frequently experience increased water loss due to medications like diuretics or increased respiratory effort, it's important to carefully monitor fluid intake and aim for adequate hydration without overloading the body. Sipping fluids throughout the day instead of consuming large amounts at once is recommended. Hydrating beverages like water, herbal teas, or diluted fruit juices are good choices. Urine color can also be used to gauge hydration levels; pale yellow indicates adequate hydration.

To maintain respiratory moisture and overall well-being, COPD patients need to maintain a balance of fluid intake that is specific to their needs and conditions. Other factors that may help with overall fluid intake include selecting foods high in water content, like fruits and vegetables, avoiding excessive caffeine and alcohol, and making sure that your home is humidified.

Herbal teas and infusions provide calming and advantageous choices for COPD sufferers seeking to manage symptoms and enhance respiratory health. Peppermint tea, for example, can ease respiratory discomfort and facilitate digestion. Chamomile tea has anti-inflammatory qualities, encouraging calmness and possibly reducing anxiety associated with respiratory problems. Ginger tea has anti-nausea qualities and can help ease respiratory congestion. All of these teas can be savored hot or cold, offering hydration in addition to their medicinal advantages.

Herbal infusions, made by adding fresh herbs like basil or thyme to hot water, can offer similar benefits with customizable flavors. Avoiding excessive sweeteners ensures the beverages retain their health benefits. Adding herbal teas and infusions to daily routines can help COPD patients manage symptoms and improve overall well-being. Making herbal teas involves steeping dried or fresh herbs in hot water for several minutes, allowing the flavors and beneficial compounds to infuse. Straining the herbs before consumption ensures a smooth texture.

RICH IN NUTRIENT SMOOTHIES

Smoothies with added protein, like protein powder or yogurt, help maintain muscle strength, which is important for respiratory support. Using liquids like water, coconut water, or almond milk ensures smooth consistency and hydration benefits. Vegetables and fruits blended allow for easy digestion and absorption of essential vitamins and minerals. Ingredients like spinach, kale, berries, and bananas provide antioxidants and fiber, supporting immune function and digestive health.

Nutrient-dense smoothies are made by blending ingredients in a blender until smooth, adding liquid to achieve the desired thickness. You can maximize the anti-inflammatory effects of omega-3 fatty acids by adding chia or flaxseeds. Drinking smoothies as a meal replacement or snack gives you sustained energy and supports respiratory function all day. You can customize your smoothies by experimenting with different ingredient combinations.

WARM DRINKS TO HELP YOU UNWIND

Warm beverages can be a source of comfort and relaxation for patients with COPD who are managing their symptoms and looking for respiratory support. Warm water with lemon boosts immune function and hydrates; herbal teas like lavender or valerian root help reduce anxiety, which can exacerbate breathing difficulties; warm milk with a dash of turmeric or cinnamon can reduce inflammation and ease respiratory passages; these drinks should be savored slowly for optimal benefits.

Warm drinks are made by heating water or milk to a comfortable temperature—boiling destroys nutritional value—and then adding natural sweeteners, such as honey or stevia, to enhance flavor without sacrificing health benefits. Warm drinks can be incorporated into daily routines, especially in the winter or right before bed, to promote respiratory comfort and relaxation. Refraining from using too much caffeine or sugar guarantees that these warm drinks promote general well-being and help manage symptoms for COPD patients.

Monitoring daily fluid intake guarantees proper hydration without surpassing the body's capacity; tracking fluid intake throughout the day, striving for consistency supports hydration levels and helps manage symptoms like mucus production and dry mouth; avoiding excessive caffeine and alcohol, which can dehydrate the body, guarantees beneficial fluids consumed. Managing fluid intake is crucial for COPD patients to maintain respiratory function and overall health.

Generally, mindful management of fluid intake tailored to individual needs enhances well-being and symptom management for COPD patients. Using tools like measured cups or water bottles with marked volumes can help track daily intake accurately. Consulting healthcare providers for personalized recommendations based on individual health needs and medications is advisable. Adapting fluid intake based on environmental factors like humidity levels or physical activity supports optimal hydration. Including hydrating foods like soups, fruits, and vegetables supplements fluid intake and supports respiratory health.

RECIPES FOR SUGAR-FREE DESSERTS

A key tactic is to swap out refined sugars for healthier alternatives to effectively manage blood sugar levels. For example, desserts can be sweetened with mashed bananas, applesauce, or dates, which provide natural sweetness and additional nutrients.

Developing low-sugar dessert recipes is crucial to continuing a COPD-friendly diet that supports overall health and well-being. These recipes emphasize minimizing added sugars while maximizing natural sweetness from ingredients like fruits or alternative sweeteners like stevia or monk fruit.

When making low-sugar desserts, it's important to strike a balance between flavors and textures without sacrificing flavor. Additives such as cocoa powder, vanilla extract, or cinnamon can intensify the sweetness without raising the sugar content. Whole grains and nuts are frequently used in recipes to add fiber and healthy fats, which support digestive health and satiety. By emphasizing nutrient-dense ingredients and clever substitutions, people with COPD can enjoy satisfying desserts without compromising their dietary goals.

Fruit-based sweets are a great choice for people with COPD because they provide natural sugars, fiber, and important vitamins. Fruit-based desserts, such as fruit salads, baked apples, or berry parfaits, bring out the sweetness of fresh fruit naturally.

Preparing fruit-based desserts is usually simple and requires little cooking to retain nutrients and flavors. For example, a basic fruit salad can have seasonal fruits with a honey drizzle or toasted almonds sprinkled on top for extra flavor and texture.

Fruit desserts can be tailored to individual preferences and dietary restrictions, such as using low-acid fruits for those who are sensitive to acidity. Serving chilled fruit-based desserts can also provide a refreshing treat during hot weather, promoting hydration and comfort. By experimenting with different fruit combinations and presentation styles, people can discover enjoyable desserts that contribute to a balanced diet-friendly for people with COPD. Fruit desserts can also provide antioxidants and anti-inflammatory properties, supporting respiratory health.

MODERATE INDULGENCE IN SWEETS

Treats like dark chocolate squares, mini cheesecakes, or individual fruit tarts can be included in a COPD diet as long as they are consumed in moderation and with an emphasis on portion control and mindful eating practices. The key is to savor each bite mindfully, appreciating the flavors and textures without going overboard. Desserts with higher-quality ingredients and lower sugar content can help manage cravings while supporting overall health goals.

When making decadent desserts, use healthier fats like avocado or coconut oil in place of butter and cream.

This will lower the amount of saturated fats while increasing the amount of beneficial nutrients. Making homemade versions allows you to control the ingredients and tailor them to your diet and the needs of managing your COPD.

By indulging in these treats on occasion and in conjunction with well-balanced meals, people can maintain a healthy relationship with food while supporting respiratory health and overall well-being.

COOLING TREATS MADE OF FROZEN FOOD

For those with COPD, frozen desserts are a great way to stay cool and still get the nutrients and hydration they need. Some examples of these treats are homemade fruit popsicles, yogurt parfaits, or fresh fruit sorbets.

These desserts can be made with natural sweeteners or a small amount of honey to satisfy your sweet tooth without going overboard. Fruit-based desserts freeze well, keeping their texture and nutritional value, so they're a great option for summertime desserts.

Simple methods like pureeing fruits with yogurt or coconut milk and freezing them in molds yield a creamy texture and allow for inventive flavor combinations like strawberry-banana or mango-coconut.

Including frozen treats in a diet for people with COPD supports hydration and can be customized to individual taste preferences and dietary restrictions. When consumed in moderation, these treats offer a cool, nutrient-rich dessert or snack that promotes comfort and satisfaction.

ADVICE FOR HAVING DESSERTS WHILE HAVING COPD

Dessert consumption with COPD requires careful selection and understanding of dietary requirements. When it comes to desserts, it's important to focus on nutrient-dense ingredients and portion control.

When desserts are included in meals instead of being eaten separately, blood sugar levels can be stabilized and energy slumps can be avoided.

Comfort when eating is ensured by selecting desserts that are easy to chew and swallow, like smooth textures or soft fruit. Drinking water or herbal teas while enjoying desserts also helps with digestion and respiratory health.

CHAPTER FOUR

BALANCED MAIN COURSES

OPTIONS FOR LEAN PROTEIN IN COPD PATIENTS

For those with COPD, selecting lean protein sources is critical because they supply vital nutrients without excess fat or sodium. Skinless chicken or turkey are good options because they are high in protein and low in saturated fats. Fish, especially omega-3 fatty fish like salmon or trout, can help lower inflammation and support lung function. Lean beef or pork cuts that have been trimmed of visible fat are also good options because they provide iron and B vitamins.

When cooking these proteins, stick to baking, grilling, or broiling techniques to minimize the amount of fat added. Use marinades made with herbs, spices, and citrus juices to boost flavor without adding more sodium. If you have COPD and find that cooking meals wear you out, cooking in larger quantities and freezing portions can help make mealtimes less stressful.

Cutting back on sodium is essential for controlling the symptoms of COPD because too much salt can make you retain fluids and make breathing harder. Instead, try seasoning food with herbs, spices, and citrus zest. Fresh herbs like rosemary, basil, and cilantro taste great and are also good for your lungs because they are high in antioxidants and anti-inflammatory qualities.

Choose whole, fresh foods over processed ones when making meal plans; include lots of fruits and vegetables (which are naturally low in sodium and high in vital vitamins and minerals); highlight high-fiber grains like quinoa or brown rice in heart-healthy recipes; and substitute healthy fats like avocado or olive oil for butter or margarine.

ONE-POT RECIPES FOR SIMPLE COOKING

For people with COPD, one-pot meals are the best option because they reduce mess and streamline the cooking process.

Look for recipes that incorporate lean proteins, whole grains, and lots of vegetables into one dish. For instance, a filling vegetable and bean soup can supply vitamins, fiber, and protein all in one easy meal. Stir-fries made with lean meats or tofu and a rainbow of colorful vegetables are easy to make and have a nutritious nutritional profile.

Investing in a slow cooker or instant pot can help you cook even easier by tenderizing tougher cuts of meat and allowing you to cook hands-off. These appliances work great for making stews, casseroles, or even oatmeal with little effort. You can save time and energy by including one-pot meals in your weekly meal plan, and you can ensure balanced nutrition to support COPD management.

PLANT-BASED AND VEGETARIAN OPTIONS

Vegetarian and plant-based diets can be a good way for COPD patients to cut back on animal products while still getting enough nutrition and supporting respiratory health.

One should make sure to include protein sources like beans, lentils, chickpeas, and tofu, as they are high in fiber, vitamins, and minerals that are vital for lung health and can also be a great way to incorporate quinoa and other whole grains as a base for nutrient-dense meals.

Examine recipes such as bean chili, grain bowls, and vegetable stir-fries; these can be tailored with a range of vibrant veggies and tasty herbs and spices.

To make things easier, make large quantities of vegetarian dishes and freeze them in portion sizes for quick and simple meals. Diets high in antioxidants and anti-inflammatory compounds can help control the symptoms of COPD and improve general health.

COOKING ADVICE FOR THOSE WITH COPD SYMPTOMS

Use lightweight cookware and utensils to reduce strain; make sure your workspace is well-ventilated to promote easier breathing; and arrange your kitchen supplies and ingredients in a way that minimizes physical exertion.

Cooking with COPD symptoms can present challenges like fatigue, shortness of breath, and limited energy.

These strategies can help people with COPD enjoy nutritious meals while minimizing the physical strain of meal preparation: plan meals in advance and enlist help from family members or caregivers when needed; use pre-cut or pre-washed fruits and vegetables to save time and effort; choose simpler recipes with fewer ingredients that require less preparation time; and prioritize resting to conserve energy.

CHAPTER FIVE

HANDLING WEIGHT SHIFTS

Small, frequent meals throughout the day can help combat fatigue and ensure adequate nutrition intake. People with COPD often experience weight changes due to factors like decreased appetite, medication side effects, and altered metabolism.

Maintaining a healthy weight is crucial for managing COPD effectively. To prevent unintended weight loss, focus on nutrient-dense foods that provide essential calories and nutrients without requiring large quantities. Meals should include lean proteins like poultry and fish, whole grains like brown rice or quinoa, and plenty of fruits and vegetables.

On the other hand, controlling weight gain can be achieved by striking a balance between the amount of calories consumed and the amount of physical activity.

To help burn calories and enhance lung function, try walking or stretching. It's also important to keep an eye on portion sizes and steer clear of processed foods high in calories. Speaking with a registered dietitian can offer individualized advice on calorie requirements and meal planning techniques specific to each person's health objectives. Individuals with COPD can benefit from a balanced diet and mindful eating habits.

HANDLING INTESTINAL PROBLEMS

For people with COPD, digestive problems like gas, bloating, and constipation can be difficult to manage. These problems are frequently made worse by medications or reduced physical activity. To help manage symptoms, include foods high in fiber, such as fruits, vegetables, and whole grains, in daily meals to encourage regular bowel movements and improve digestive health. Drinking plenty of fluids, especially water, helps soften stools and prevent dehydration, which can exacerbate constipation.

All things considered, managing digestive issues associated with COPD can be achieved with a balanced diet that supports digestive health and by avoiding trigger foods (such as carbonated beverages and high-fat meals) that contribute to bloating or discomfort. Eating smaller, more frequent meals instead of large portions can also ease digestion and prevent discomfort after eating. Probiotics-rich foods, like yogurt or kefir, can help maintain healthy gut flora and aid digestion.

MANAGING SENSITIVITIES AND FOOD ALLERGIES

Food allergies and sensitivities can make dietary decisions more difficult for people with COPD, affecting both respiratory symptoms and general health. Identifying allergens through allergy testing or food diaries can help identify trigger foods. If sensitivities are found, common allergens like dairy, gluten, or nuts should be avoided. Carefully reading food labels and informing restaurant staff of dietary restrictions can prevent unintentional exposure to allergens and lower the risk of allergic reactions.

To maintain optimal health and effectively manage COPD symptoms, it is important to replace allergenic foods with suitable alternatives that can ensure balanced nutrition without compromising dietary needs. For example, dairy-free alternatives like almond milk or soy yogurt can replace traditional dairy products. Additionally, focusing on fresh, whole foods and cooking at home can help lower the risk of allergen contamination.

Finally, seeking advice from a healthcare provider or allergist regarding the management of food allergies and incorporating safe substitutes into daily meals is crucial.

KEEPING A HEALTHY DIET DURING SYMPTOMS

Maintaining adequate nutrition is essential during COPD exacerbations to support immune function and aid in recovery; however, eating can be difficult due to decreased appetite, fatigue, and increased difficulty breathing. Eating smaller, more frequent meals that are easy to chew and swallow can help conserve energy and reduce discomfort.

Nutrient-rich foods, like soups, smoothies, and soft fruits, can provide essential vitamins and minerals without requiring a lot of work.

Staying adequately hydrated is also important to prevent dehydration and thin mucus secretions, which makes breathing easier. It is imperative to closely monitor weight changes and symptoms and to seek medical attention as soon as possible if eating difficulties persist.

ADVICE ON EATING OUT WHILE HAVING COPD

Dining out can provide logistical challenges for people with COPD, including figuring out restaurant menus, controlling portion sizes, and making sure dietary restrictions are followed.

Selecting eateries that serve lighter fare, like grilled or steamed dishes, can help cut down on excess fat and sodium intake. Asking for accommodations, like extra sauces or dressings on the side, allows for better control over portion sizes and dietary preferences.

To make dining out more comfortable, check online menus or call ahead to ask about allergens or special dietary requirements. Bringing prescription medications or rescue inhalers ensures that you're ready for any unexpected respiratory symptoms.

CHAPTER SIX

LIFESTYLE SUGGESTIONS FOR THE MANAGEMENT OF COPD

REGULAR PHYSICAL ACTIVITY IS ESSENTIAL

Maintaining a regular physical activity schedule is critical to the successful management of COPD. Exercises that target lung function and overall endurance can improve lung function and quality of life for COPD patients. Aerobic exercises, like cycling, walking, and swimming, strengthen respiratory muscles and improve cardiovascular health. They also improve oxygen circulation throughout the body, which is critical for lowering symptoms like dyspnea. Strength training exercises further improve muscle tone and endurance, reducing the strain of daily activities.

Before beginning any physical activity, it is important to speak with a healthcare provider about your fitness level and the severity of your COPD. Start with gentle activities and work your way up to more intense ones as your endurance improves. Breathing techniques, like pursed-lip breathing and diaphragmatic breathing, can help you manage breathlessness during exercise. Monitoring your heart rate and oxygen levels during your workouts ensures safety and maximum benefit. In general, incorporating regular physical activity into daily routines not only supports physical health but also improves mood and reduces stress related to managing your COPD.

TECHNIQUES FOR STRESS MANAGEMENT

To improve overall well-being and manage symptoms, patients with COPD must learn to manage their stress. Prolonged stress can worsen symptoms and negatively affect lung function.

Deep breathing exercises, progressive muscle relaxation, and mindfulness meditation are effective ways to reduce anxiety and promote relaxation, which can ease symptoms like fatigue and shortness of breath. Including regular relaxation exercises, like yoga or guided imagery can also help patients feel calmer and develop better-coping mechanisms in stressful situations.

Establishing a stress-free environment at home entails setting priorities for self-care activities such as hobbies, socializing with supportive friends and family, and engaging in enjoyable activities; learning to delegate tasks and seeking support from loved ones can also help to reduce stress; joining support groups or counseling sessions specifically designed for COPD patients offers a forum for sharing experiences and learning practical coping strategies from peers facing similar challenges; and finally, by integrating stress management techniques into daily routines, COPD patients can improve overall quality of life and emotional resilience.

ENHANCING THE QUALITY OF SLEEP

Good sleep hygiene is promoted by establishing a regular sleep schedule and developing a relaxing bedtime routine. This includes avoiding stimulants like caffeine and nicotine close to bedtime and creating a comfortable sleep environment with proper ventilation and minimal noise disruptions. For COPD patients, getting enough sleep is essential to optimizing health outcomes and managing symptoms effectively.

Monitoring medication effects on sleep patterns is important, as some medications used to manage COPD symptoms may affect sleep quality. Breathing exercises, like pursed-lip breathing, before bedtime can help relax the airways and improve the quality of sleep. Elevating the head with pillows or using a wedge pillow supports better breathing and reduces discomfort during sleep. Practicing relaxation techniques, like progressive muscle relaxation or guided imagery can calm the mind and prepare the body for restful sleep.

Regular daytime physical activity improves sleep patterns and general health. However, intense exercise should be avoided right before bed as it may prevent you from falling asleep. COPD patients can improve their quality of sleep, improve their daytime functioning, and better manage their condition's symptoms by emphasizing sleep hygiene practices and incorporating relaxation techniques into their daily routines.

SUPPORT FOR QUITTING SMOKING

One of the most crucial things COPD patients can do to slow down the progression of their disease and enhance their overall health is to stop smoking. To help patients quit, smoking cessation support services include creating a customized plan that includes identifying triggers, setting a date for quitting, and getting professional advice from healthcare providers or cessation counselors. Nicotine replacement therapies, like patches or gum, can help manage cravings and withdrawal symptoms that come with stopping smoking.

A smoke-free home and avoiding situations where smoking is common to support long-term success in quitting. COPD patients are more likely to commit to their quitting journey when they are aware of the health benefits of quitting, such as improved lung function and reduced risk of disease complications.

Participating in behavioral counseling or support groups designed specifically for smoking cessation offers emotional support and strategies to overcome challenges during the quitting process.

Healthy coping strategies, like exercise and stress reduction, help control cravings and lessen the impulse to smoke. Marking progress and accomplishments along the way encourages positive behavior changes and increases self-esteem. Patients with COPD can greatly enhance their quality of life, respiratory health, and general well-being by committing to quitting smoking and making use of the support services that are available to them.

ADVICE FOR KEEPING A POSITIVE ATTITUDE

Remaining optimistic is crucial for managing COPD and enhancing quality of life. Setting reasonable objectives and acknowledging accomplishments, no matter how minor, can increase motivation and self-worth. Indulging in joyful and fulfilling activities, like hobbies or quality time with loved ones, can improve emotional health. Being grateful and living in the present moment can help divert attention from negative thoughts and foster a positive outlook. Seeking support from medical professionals, therapists, or support groups can offer support and direction during trying times. Resilience and optimism in adjusting to life changes can help people with COPD face obstacles head-on.

CHAPTER SEVEN

TAKING CARE OF NUTRITIONAL ISSUES IN COPD

Maintaining a balanced diet is essential for individuals with COPD to support overall respiratory function and energy levels. Key nutritional concerns include managing weight fluctuations, ensuring adequate intake of essential nutrients, and addressing potential dietary restrictions or sensitivities. Nutrition plays a crucial role in managing COPD (Chronic Obstructive Pulmonary Disease), focusing on maintaining optimal health and managing symptoms effectively.

Nutrient-dense foods like fruits, vegetables, whole grains, and lean proteins are often the focus of a COPD-friendly diet. These foods offer vital vitamins, minerals, and antioxidants that support lung health and general well-being. Patients with COPD are also advised to watch how much sodium they consume to control fluid retention and preserve cardiovascular health.

Adequate hydration is also stressed to help thin mucus secretions, which facilitates clearing the airways.

Additionally, calorie requirements might differ depending on the severity of the disease and individual factors. For example, some patients might need more calories to maintain their energy levels, while others might need to prioritize nutrient density to prevent excessive weight gain. Speaking with a registered dietitian can assist in creating a customized nutrition plan that addresses specific COPD-related concerns while also meeting individual needs.

FAQS REGARDING DIETARY CHANGES

Changing eating habits is a common concern for people with COPD. Common questions center around doable strategies for controlling symptoms with diet. For example, patients frequently ask about the function of carbohydrates in sustaining energy levels and how to include them without aggravating symptoms like gas or bloating. Another common question is about the effects of fats and selecting healthier options like omega-3 fatty acids, as these fats can help reduce inflammation in the body.

Intake of protein is also important because it supports respiratory health and muscle strength; many patients ask for advice on easy-to-digest protein sources that are low in saturated fats. Questions about particular vitamins and minerals, such as magnesium and vitamin D, come up because of their roles in immune system support and maintaining muscle health, which are critical for managing COPD.

Lastly, patients frequently inquire about the role of supplements in their diet, such as antioxidants or herbal remedies, to complement their nutritional intake and support overall lung health.

Managing fluid intake is a concern, especially for patients with fluid retention issues. It can be difficult to balance hydration needs while avoiding excessive intake. Patients frequently ask these questions.

For COPD patients, meal preparation can be made easier by emphasizing nutritious, quick-to-prepare meals that promote respiratory health. Some helpful hints include planning to minimize effort when feeling exhausted or having trouble breathing, and cooking meals in bulk that can be frozen for later use to guarantee that there are healthy options available without requiring a lot of cooking every day.

Selecting recipes that call for the least amount of prep and cooking time is advantageous. For instance, going with easy stir-fries or salads with pre-cut veggies and lean proteins saves energy and cooking time. Using kitchen appliances such as pressure cookers or slow cookers can also streamline meal preparation by reducing the amount of time spent cooking by hand.

Additionally, including COPD-friendly snacks like nuts, yogurt, or fresh fruits can help sustain energy levels between meals without causing discomfort. Portion control is crucial to avoid overeating, which can result in bloating or increased effort required to breathe. In summary, implementing a meal planning strategy that strikes a balance between practicality and nutritional requirements can promote the best possible health and well-being for people with COPD.

HANDLING SHIFTS IN APPETITE

Patients with COPD frequently experience changes in appetite as a result of medication side effects, decreased physical activity, or changes in their sense of taste or smell. One coping strategy is to eat smaller, more frequent meals throughout the day to avoid feeling full or uncomfortable.

Patients are also encouraged to concentrate on nutrient-dense foods that offer vital vitamins and minerals without being overly caloric.

To address taste changes, one way to improve flavor is to experiment with herbs, spices, or marinades instead of using too much salt or sugar. Another way to help patients who have trouble swallowing or with their teeth are to choose foods that are easier to chew and swallow. Lastly, adding different textures to meals—such as soft meats or crunchy vegetables—can increase appetite and make eating more pleasurable.

Keeping a food diary can help track intake patterns and identify triggers for appetite fluctuations, allowing for necessary adjustments to meal planning and preparation. Watching weight changes is important for both patients and caregivers and if significant appetite changes persist, consulting with a healthcare provider or dietitian is advised.

ADVICE FOR COPD PATIENTS REGARDING SUPPLEMENTS

Vitamin D supplementation is often advised due to its role in immune function and bone health, especially for individuals who may have limited sun exposure. Omega-3 fatty acids, which help reduce inflammation and support cardiovascular health, are among the supplements that are frequently recommended for COPD patients to complement their diet and support overall health.

As they help fight oxidative stress and inflammation in the lungs, antioxidant supplements like vitamin C or E may also be helpful. However, it's important to speak with a healthcare professional before beginning any new supplement regimen because some supplements may interact with medications or make preexisting conditions worse.

In addition, individuals with COPD should exercise caution when using herbal supplements and seek advice from a pharmacist or healthcare provider to guarantee safety and efficacy. Certain herbal remedies have the potential to interact with medications or worsen respiratory symptoms. In general, supplement use should be customized to the patient's specific needs and supervised by medical professionals to maximize benefits and minimize risks.